Love and Greed That Kill

Love and Greed That Kill

How Plant Poisoning Is Covertly Being Portrayed as Voodoo

Lillian Burton

ISBN: **1518737234**
ISBN **13: 9781518737237**
Library of Congress Control Number: **2015920452**
CreateSpace Independent Publishing Platform
North Charleston, SC

Contents

Conclusion

References

Preface

I have always been a very opinionated person. I believe in thinking and doing for myself. I believe in doing what I think is feasible to help others, and I believe that people need to help themselves instead of relying on others to do everything for them. My reasons for doing the research required to write this book are numerous. I was raised from the age of six weeks to an adult by my paternal grandmother, someone whom I still love and adore as my mother. Once, I witnessed her experience a severe case of gastritis. Her doctors could not determine the source of her illness.

After being married for approximately twenty-six years, I experienced a rise in blood pressure from overactive adrenal glands from an unknown cause.

Another incident occurred during my teaching career while I was sitting in the middle-school cafeteria having lunch with my class. I overheard a conversation among a certain group of teachers from a nearby table bragging about how to secretly feed people to force them into doing anything you want them to do. I thought that was strange and impossible.

At other times, I have found in my home weird-looking solutions in Ziploc bags and in other containers hidden in the attic down in the fiberglass insulation.

Lastly, I had the experience of taking a very close family member to dinner to help console her in the recent loss of her husband. While we were having dinner, I went to the ladies' room. While I was in the ladies' room, she slipped something in my water. When I returned to my dinner, I was very lucky to be able to detect the bitter, flat taste. I asked her about it; she lied and said it was the taste of the water from the restaurant. I was perplexed, because it did not have that taste before I went to the ladies' room.

I have seen otherwise healthy people who either were having a marital affair or were financially comfortable suddenly become ill and die, with doctors puzzled about the cause of their illness and sudden death.

8

I knew from growing up in rural northern Mississippi that something strange was practiced by certain families that was called voodoo, and you were cautioned to stay away from those families and not eat anything they offered to you. You should eat at home. After all my experiences and those of others, I decided to research what some were referring to as voodoo, because I knew that voodoo is a religion, and I could not understand the consciousness of doing evil to people in the name of religion. I wanted to find out what plant sources are used, what toxins are in the plants, and what autoimmune diseases they create. I want people, especially medical professionals and law-enforcement officials, to be cognizant of how plant poisoning and in some cases animal poisoning are being referred to as voodoo, but are actually tools manufactured and sold on the black market to control people. What voodoo practitioners are really doing is torturing and murdering innocent people.

Introduction

Mild hypertension had always been a part of my life, since my early teenage years, but it was never severe enough to require medication. However, years after I grew up, my grandmother became weak and needed the attention of a nursing home. This sudden change caused me to become dependent on blood-pressure medicine, one pill daily. This continued for approximately fifteen years. Getting the proper exercise, eating correctly, and getting an annual physical were parts of my routine in an effort to maintain my health.

As time progressed, my internist noticed that my blood pressure had suddenly become elevated. Medications were added to remedy my blood pressure. This worked for a while, but then it continued to increase. More medications were added. Tests were conducted, but there was no physical reason for its occurrence. My internist asked me if I was eating a lot of licorice candy, to which I replied no, because I hate that flavor. I was referred to an endocrinologist, who conducted tests that revealed that too much aldosterone was being produced by my adrenal glands. Somehow, they had suddenly become hyperactive. The recommendation was to remove the left adrenal gland. Once my left adrenal gland was removed, my blood pressure returned to normal. During my postoperative period, it remained normal. But after I returned to my classroom duties as a science teacher, somehow my blood pressure began to increase again—even though I loved and enjoyed teaching, as well as my students.

There were periods of confusion and dizziness that I had cast aside as typical fatigue. I had begun to have noticeable problems with my memory that I did not tell anyone about. I could not remember mathematical facts long enough to walk from my desk over to a student's desk or over to the chalkboard to demonstrate scientific or mathematical solutions to my students. I could not remember telephone numbers, which was something I had been able to do for long periods of time. When I approached traffic intersections, I was having problems determining what to do. I had to concentrate extremely hard to determine if I needed to stop or go. I noticed that I had also developed a bitter palate. All of this made me wonder what was happening to me.

One day I was teaching my high-school chemistry class when one of my female students came over to me. She took my left wrist as she said to me, "Come here and let me show you something." She led me to her desk to view some work she had completed and wanted me to critique. When she grabbed my wrist, it felt strange, so I looked down at both my wrists. They were both swollen; my knees were slightly swollen too.

When I was at home, I would sip on a Diet Coke all day because I did not normally drink an entire twelve-ounce can during a meal. I began to notice a bitter taste in my leftover Diet Cokes. I stated to a family member, "Someone is putting something in my Cokes!" My family member replied, "No, that's all that medicine you are taking." The arguments became very heated, and the family split.

I went to my doctor and explained to him that I thought I had been poisoned. He prescribed steroids, which resolved most of the swelling. I had a toxicology test done on my urine at a nearby lab. The results were normal. However, lab personnel informed me that I had waited too long before getting my sample to them, because some drugs metabolize quicker than others.

I knew from growing up in my neighborhood that there were people who were afraid of certain families because they had a reputation for practicing hoodoo, which is often referred to as voodoo. I never believed it because of the way it was practiced at the time.

My purpose for writing this book is to reveal several things. I will first give some history of voodoo, specifically how voodoo-hoodoo was practiced before the twentieth century as opposed to how it is being practiced in 2015. Then, I will explain how plant poisoning is erroneously being referred to as voodoo, and how plant poisoning is related to certain autoimmune diseases. Finally, I will explain how plant poisoning is flowing on the black market.

Chapter 1

Voodoo/Hoodoo History

During the 1700s, some African slaves were sold to the West Indies before their arrival in the United States. While there, their method of practicing their religion was called voodoo. The word initially began as *vodu*, but through a series of changes, it slowly became *voodoo*. According to Tallant (1946), the name has been corrupted down through the years and incorrect enunciation the word hoodoo was used and is still pronounced as such.

African slave voodoo involved rites and customs such as snake worshipping and dancing. They worked in chains, heavily guarded, from sunrise to sunset. They were locked in guarded quarters at night. They experienced problems practicing their religion because they were forbidden by their slave owners. Slave owners restricted their ceremonies because they were in constant fear of an uprising, since they were outnumbered by slaves. There were some slave owners who allowed their slaves to assemble to practice their religion and to have ritual dances. However, if the slave owners were caught allowing this practice, they were assessed a fine and had to make a payment of crowns to the treasury of the church for the first offense. The second offense of the slave owner would require a lifetime of working in the king's galleys. Blacks who were caught were whipped.

Once the blacks arrived as slaves in the United States in New Orleans, Louisiana, they were still forbidden to hold their religious ceremonies. To remedy this, the slaves did a phony conversion to Catholicism so they could assemble. After Louisiana was purchased by the United States from France in 1803, there were second and third generations of slaves whose attitudes and personalities had mellowed. They could speak the English language and did not have any past memory of the cruel treatment by slave owners. The prohibition against African slaves of the West Indies had been removed. A huge population of free blacks from the West Indies came to New Orleans, and voodoo began to be practiced openly.

The voodoo ceremonies were held late at night, and they had a queen and sometimes a king who was not always present at the ceremonies. The king was usually the current lover of the queen. Items used in their ceremonies included drums, erotic dancing, bonfires, snakes, sacrifices, gris-gris (pronounced as gray-gray), a black cat, a rooster, a bowl of blood from the kid of a goat, and alcoholic beverages. They had incense and holy water that had been adopted from Catholicism. Gris-gris were dolls made of feathers, hair, snakeskin, and pieces of human bones, and they sometimes had a black-cat bone stuffed inside. The queen would also be referred to as a priestess.

During their ceremonial activities, the priestess would use a snake (usually a python) during her dance, which was in a circle. She would lift the snake close to her face. If the snake licked her cheek that would make her an oracle, which was believed to give her the power to see visions. It was also believed that she could make predictions about someone's future and interpret signs.

The queen during the early 1800s in New Orleans was Marie Laveau. Her ceremonies were a little different. She had not only snakes, a black cat, and rooster-blood drinking, but also a lot of fornication, Roman Catholic statues, prayers, incense, holy water, and guinea peppers. She added tricks of her own to her ceremonies. She combined elements of Catholicism with voodoo, and, according to Tallant (1946), she implemented plant poisoning in her voodoo business. Depending on who was talking, she was either a ruthless witch or a saint.

During her ceremonies, the music would begin slow and then become wild. There would be a pot of water hanging over an open fire where members would toss in their offerings. The sacrifices would be such things as chickens, cats, frogs, snakes, and other small animals that they would drop in the pot of boiling water. After the offering, a male dancer dressed in loincloth would appear in the center holding a baby-sized coffin, while other members were chanting. He would place the coffin at the feet of the queen and continue to whirl around in his dance until he fell to the ground from exhaustion. Other members would continue to dance and drink from the pot. They would also drink a product called tafia (moonshine whiskey). Tallant (1946) also indicated that white children were used in sacrifices. Queens were often accused of kidnapping and murdering white children. Years later they began to eat gumbo, cooked chicken, and guzzle alcohol during their ceremonies.

During some ceremonies on the shore of Lake Pontchartrain, the queen would be wearing a few handkerchiefs on a cord around her body as she danced erotically. The other females would wear the same attire, but mostly of a different color. The males would wear loincloths. Certain indoor ceremonies involved one young lady in the center of the circle, wearing a thin nightgown with more than one hundred males dancing around her. In the room was a pot cooking that included snakes and frogs. This was done to regain the affection of a man she loved. Chicken, cake, and rum were served. The Creole dance involved wearing ankle bells and knee rings as musical instruments. The dance would begin with one man dancing with two women. They wore knee rings that made music as they danced. They would eat and drink some type of alcoholic beverage. When the queen yelled out a signal, everyone stripped off their handkerchiefs and loincloths and jumped into the lake. There were instances in which some were so drunk that they drowned.

In the community the queen was a flamboyantly dressed, free woman of color. When she walked down the streets of New Orleans, there would be a crowd following her. She invited everyone to her ceremonies, although there were ceremonies not everyone knew about. Her ceremonies were heavily attended by whites. White women joined the voodoo sect mostly for the fun. White men attended because they were interested not only in the fun but they were also interested in dating the mulatto and black women. White men and mulatto women would dance naked all night long.

Marie Laveau was successful in making predictions and telling fortunes, because she was a hairdresser to mulatto and white women. She had people hired who were employed in the homes of wealthy people and could bring her gossip. They would reveal to her personal family business of their employers. When her clients came to her for advice, they were often amazed that she could tell them secrets about their own personal lives.

Many marriages among whites were for business arrangements. Wealthy men had beautiful mistresses (mulatto and black women) living in nearby cottages. Marie Laveau was also successful because she would attack other queens and drive them from the area. She would go out late at night and leave dolls with a pin inserted or a wax ball covered with feathers on the doorsteps of certain black women in the neighborhood that worked in wealthy homes. The next morning after the black women had seen the strange items, they would come to Queen Marie asking for help in removing the spirit.

Queen Marie was Roman Catholic. Some research indicates that she had fifteen children by her husband, while other research states that her children had different fathers. Some of her children died at a young age, and some lived to become adults. She also had siblings, believed to have practiced voodoo as well, who had moved away from New Orleans to other parts of the United States. There have been several Marie Laveaus. It has been speculated that the family consisted of a dynasty. During her life she displayed two different personalities. To some she was an awful, old voodoo woman, and to others she was an angel. When one of her daughters became Marie I, she was referred to as the Widow Paris. She had lived with several husbands, but Paris was one of the first two. In her later years, she changed her ways and began to give care and assistance to victims during the yellow-fever epidemic. She died a devout Catholic at the approximate age of eighty-five.

According to Tallant (1946), the voodoo religion has been characterized as an "easy love, easy money" maker, because it is the smartest racket in the world. In the early 1900s, law enforcement began to crack down on voodoo practitioners because they were swindling people and causing harm to clients due to improper health practices. They were selling false hope just to get the money.

Voodoo practitioners often used a certain plant, five-finger grass in its dried, crushed form. Each leaf point was said to bring luck in a given area: luck, money, wisdom, power, or love. This plant is actually cinquefoil or European five-finger grass, an herb that has medicinal uses for the skin. It has tannins that are astringents, which are skin-drying agents. Proper dosage had not been established for safe health usage. In 1940 it was sold for $0.25; now in 2015, its online prices range from $2.00 to $11.00 depending on the amount purchased.

Research has indicated that Queen Marie Laveau sacrificed children and helped women kill unwanted babies. There were implications that some queens provided poison to their clients to kill people when there was feuding among people in a neighborhood. When a person from one group was given a poison, became ill, and died, the revenge was to extend the same favor by poisoning a member of the opposing group. There is a lot of research about root work and healing with the use of herbs, but I was unable to find evidence of this in the research where poisoning was used in voodoo before Queen Laveau's reign. According to Tallant (1946), people in New Orleans were poisoned with vegetable salads.

Medical professionals and law enforcement have been unable to take action in the past, because they had no knowledge or idea of what was wrong with their patients. Doctors in Louisiana were often mystified and could not ascertain the causes of certain illnesses or deaths. There were no toxicology tests or screenings available. Of course, if you listen to your body, you can often determine when you have been given something weird.

The next section will address the relationship between voodoo and plant poisoning. Voodoo is still in practice today, and some groups are actually having ceremonies without using plant poisoning. But other groups are in the practice of secretly administering plant poisoning to others. No ceremonies are held by the latter; it is on the black market, only by word of mouth.

Chapter 2

Plant Sources

The toxic cocktails or toxic teas that they create will be determined by what they have available—those plants are going to be what they have or can plant in their homes, yards, or flower gardens. It is their means of self-employment, and they will use plants that can be easily obtained from garden centers at Home Depot, Lowes, Walmart, and other local nurseries or that can be ordered online. In the process of doing my research, I was able to find 112 plants that are growing in the wild as well as around and inside the home. With populations increasing in cities and decreasing in rural areas, home poison manufacturers are going to use what is cheap, convenient, and easily accessible. The makers and sellers of plant poisoning usually grow their own plants from purchasing seeds and small plants. These individuals will specialize in creating their product with three or four plants, but sometimes it may be as few as one or two plants. Criminals do not tell their poison-making secrets to just anyone. They only share their little secret with trusted family and friends, because it is a business. It is all about getting as much tax-free income as possible. Therefore, most people are not aware of how it is done. They think it is some special God-given gift or talent that only certain people have. The criminals market their products by word of mouth. They seek out people who are always complaining. People who manufacture and sell plant poison will look for clients who meet certain criteria. Their clients are gainfully employed. They are unhappy people who think everything should go their way. They have become very angry. Their clients will often have personal family issues, such as a spouse or other family member with problems of alcoholism, or infidelity. They will also have clients who have problems on their jobs, not able to perform and in possible danger of losing a job or cannot get that promotion, and decides to use plant poison to move that person out of their path to achieving what they desire. Clients also want to force other people to give them what they want. Poison makers will approach their potential clients in a friendly manner, often in public places. They will talk to them long enough to pick their brains to find out what problems or desires they have that can be capitalized on. They will then use that knowledge of problems to promote their products. Sometimes plant poisoning is market by day and sold after dark, at night. They have their clients come by their homes at night to buy the poison. It is usually in liquid form to be infused in the victim's beverage or dinner. After a certain level of trust has developed between the poison maker and the client the exchange of poison and money can be made anywhere and at any time. Their dispensing containers are often recycled. They sell the poison in volume containers. The amount of liquid toxic tea requested will determine the size of the container. Large amounts, gallons, are sold in old pickle jars, the one-hundred-twenty-eight-ounce size. Smaller amounts are sold in quart, pint, and smaller-ounce-size containers that may be glass or plastic. The smaller-ounce-size bottles will range from one-half ounce to as much as three-and-one-half-ounce sizes. Clients will hide this poison in the attic within the fiberglass insulation, in a kitchen cabinet, in a locked outdoor shed, or even in a locked vehicle. Where it is hidden depends on what other family members are living in the home, their awareness of the plant poisoning, and the intended victim. When the criminal decides to administer the poison to someone outside of the home, the poison is carried in their personal pocket or inside of a ladies' purse. The container at this point will be a small bottle that resembles an ornamental fingernail polish, perfume, or cologne bottle and can hold as much as one-half to one ounce of liquid. They will also use sandwich-size Ziploc bags to transport it to use on their victim. The bottles are in a variety of colors. Some are ornamental with an antique look. I have seen one in a kitchen cabinet in an emerald-green glass bottle that could hold approximately three ounces. The appearance of the toxic tea is determined by the plants and the parts used. Its appearance can range from the looks of green tea, cinnamon tea, or dirty car-wash water to a thin milky-white color with black particles suspended in it.

After the product has been swallowed by the victim the criminal or purchaser of the poisonous potion will ask for what is desired from the victim. If the victim is a spouse, they will watch to see if that philandering spouse has fallen asleep. Why? So the spouse will be unable to go out, to get a drink, or to become abusive. Depending on how many times the poison has been administered to the spouse, he or she will possibly be too ill to be abusive anymore or can suddenly fall dead.

When victims go to their physicians for help with the illness, the medical professional provides help based on his or her professional training and information provided by the patient. The criminal gets away because the poisoning goes undetected. Toxicology screening is not conducted. Lantadene poisoning is usually diagnosed as a drinking problem because an otherwise healthy individual who enjoys an occasional drink has suddenly developed liver disease. A person suddenly develops psychosis after being fed the Ergot toxin, but test results may show traces of LSD. Physicians will think drug use. Criminals are getting away with physiological abuse with the intent to murder, mental abuse, torture, and murder.

Chapter 3

Avoiding Plant Poisoning

If you suspect that you have been given a poison, please seek the help of a medical professional and inform him or her that you think you have been clandestinely given a poison. If you have any of the remaining contents of what you were given, take it with you to your nearest emergency room or medical doctor. The medical professional should contact the poison-control center at 1-800-222-1212. It would be helpful to keep activated charcoal in your medicine cabinet, because this will absorb any poison remaining in the stomach. It must be taken as soon as possible after the poison has been swallowed. It will not help if too much time has passed, because some of the poison may have been metabolized by the liver and gone to other parts of the body. If you are fortunate enough to survive a poisoning event and you did not seek the care of a physician, you still need to detox your body. Ask your doctor to recommend a good product for you, since he or she is aware of your health history.

There may be some in your circle who are hateful, envious, or full of greed, and who are out to get you. So, if you decide to press your luck and enjoy the fellowship of others at a private party, potluck dinner, church dinner, or other event in someone else's home, be careful, because the ones you think you can trust may be the ones that you discover you cannot. If you need to leave your food, you need to do one of three things: (1) try to eat what you want before leaving, (2) if possible, take your food with you, or (3) order a replacement. Of course, it's safest to eat alone. At church dinners, private parties, or privately held banquet dinners, you should exercise extreme caution. Food that has been specially prepared for you should only be eaten if the cook is eating with you. Prepare your own plate while the host or hostess is preparing his or hers. Save some (in a doggie bag) to take home with you in case you have delayed illness. You will have saved your evidence! Any food the host is not eating you should bypass as well. People will eat their own cooking, but they will not eat their own cooking if it contains a poison. If it is not suitable for them to eat, leave it, because it is certainly not suitable for you. Again, leave it!

Chapter 4

Plant Poisoning

Plant poisoning has been practiced at least since the days of Socrates, around 399 BC. He was a person who questioned everything, and he taught his students this attitude as well. The Athenians did not like this and believed he was spoiling the youth. He suffered a lot for this. He had the opportunity to leave the situation but chose to stay. He was given hemlock poisoning, which caused his death (Stewart 2009; Püssa 2014).

Plant poisoning was used during trials in which the accused were forced to drink a poisonous tea. The belief was that if you vomited the concoction or if you survived the ordeal, you were innocent, but if you died, you were guilty. People practicing plant poisoning today are using a similar thought process. They have the brainless belief that if you are deliberately fed poison (their blessed water), you will grant them anything they wish from you. The reasons are usually to control an abusive or cheating spouse or to loosen up a tightfisted spouse or other family member, close friend, or anyone they can think of that can promote their cause.

When people are out to get you, it is often hard to determine which plants they have used. Home manufacturers, people who make or cook the toxic cocktails and teas, are hustling. They are only interested in the large sums of tax-free income that they are able to earn on the black market by selling these products to those who are ignorant and yearning to control or get even with someone.

Different plants present different problems, because they have different toxins and belong to different plant families. I have organized plants according to families, toxins, and the symptoms that can result. The symptoms usually reveal themselves based on how much is ingested (Turner and von Aderkas 2009; Wink and van Wyk 2008; and Stewart 2009).

Arum and Grape families have related toxins		
Arum Family		
Plant	Toxin	Symptom
Elephant ears, alocasias, or taros, anthuriums, arums, Italian lords and ladies, cuckoo plant, Caladiums, calla lily, dumbcanes, philodendrons, monsteras, Jack-in-the-pulpit, Eastern skunk cabbage, Western skunk cabbage, and water arum.	Calcium oxalate in the entire plant.	Contact irritation of skin and eyes. Painful irritation and swelling of lips, mouth, and throat.
Grape Family		
Plant	Toxin	Symptom
Virginia creeper	Calcium oxalate crystals	Irritation and swelling of the skin, eyes, mouth, and tongue. Other symptoms include nausea, vomiting, diarrhea, and feelings of the urgent need to urinate or have a bowel movement.
Buckwheat Family		
Plant	Toxin	Symptom
Rhubarb	Calcium oxalate	Irritation and swelling of the

		skin, eyes, mouth, and tongue. Other symptoms include nausea, vomiting, diarrhea, and feelings of the urgent need to urinate or have a bowel movement.

In addition to symptoms listed in the chart, anthuriums will also cause difficulty in swallowing, loss of speech, and loss of appetite. Dumbcanes will also cause lots of salivation, swelling of the throat (which may lead to choking), nausea, vomiting, and diarrhea. On rare occasions Jack-in-the-pulpit, Eastern skunk cabbage, Western skunk cabbage, and water arum, can cause an irregular heartbeat, dilated pupils, coma, and death.

Rhubarb belongs to the buckwheat family, but I have included it with the arum family because it contains calcium oxalic. The toxin is in all parts of the plant except its leaves. Toxic dosage will cause severe abdominal pain, difficulty breathing, drowsiness, and muscle twitching in addition to all of the above-mentioned symptoms. Poisoning from it may be hard to detect because symptoms are delayed for as long as one hour.

Aster and Borage families consist of similar toxins		
Aster Family		
Plant	Toxin	Symptom
Cocklebur	Carboxyatractyloside	Loss of appetite, inflammation of the digestive tract, excitability, weakness, loss of coordination, prostration, convulsion, and death
White snakeroot, stinking chamomile, stinking maywood, tasselflower, brickel bush, yellow star-thistle, tarbush, blackbrush, sneezeweed, snakeweed, rubberweed, copperweed, paperflower, cutleaf, coneflower, glow wort, goldenrod, common tansy,	Tremetol in the entire plant	Weakness, difficulty walking, salivation, nausea, vomiting, loss of appetite, labored breathing, tremors, jaundice, constipation, prostration, delirium, and, in severe cases, death.

horsebrush, ragwort, and rough cocklebur		
Tansy ragwort	Senecionine, seneciphylline, jaconine, and jacobine. Toxins are carcinogenic.	Abdominal pain, nausea, vomiting, headache, enlarged liver, apathy, emaciation, and liver damage
Borage Family		
Plant	Toxin	Symptom
Heliotropes, comfreys, gypsyflower, viper's buglosses, and fiddlenecks	Senecionine, seneciphylline, jaconine, and jacobine	Abdominal pain, nausea, vomiting, headache, enlarged liver, apathy, and emaciation.

Barberry Family		
Plant	Toxin	Symptom
Mayapple	Lignans podophyllin, alpha- and beta-peltatin, in the entire plant	Touching rhizomes can cause skin and eye irritation, keratitis, and ulcerative skin lesions. Ingesting causes severe vomiting and diarrhea, blood abnormalities, kidney failure, and eventual coma.

Beech Family		
Plant	Toxin	Symptom
Oregon white oak, Garry oak, white oak, and red oak	Ellagitannin, proanthocyanidin, and gallotannins in the young shoots, acorns, and foliage	Raw, untreated acorns cause painful and lingering irritation of the mouth and throat; inflammation, irritation, and hemorrhaging of the intestinal walls; and degeneration of the liver and kidneys.

Bittersweet Family		
Plant	Toxin	Symptom
Burning bush and spindle trees	Digitaloids, aglycone, several peptides, and sesquiterpene alkaloids	Watery diarrhea, persistent vomiting, fever, chills, weakness, hallucinations, convulsions, and coma.

Boxwood Family		
Plant	Toxin	Symptom
Common box plant	buxines	Abdominal pain, vomiting, and diarrhea. Large doses cause lack of coordination, convulsions, coma, and death from respiratory failure.

Buckeye and Horse Chestnut families have similar toxins		
Buckeye Family		
Plant	Toxin	Symptom
Buckeyes	Aescin	Weakness, loss of coordination, vomiting, twitching, dilated pupils, sluggishness, excitability, and paralysis
Horse Chestnut Family		
Plant	Toxin	Symptom
Horse chestnut	Aescin	Inflammation of the mucous membranes, thirst, vomiting, weakness, lack of coordination, muscle twitching, dilated pupils, stupor, paralysis, coma, and death from respiratory paralysis

Buckthorn Family		
Plant	Toxin	Symptom
Coyotillo	Neurotoxins including anthracenes, a naphthalene derivative	Weakness, lack of coordination, and complete collapse, followed by paralysis that may be delayed from a few days to as long as several weeks

Buttercup, Ginseng, and Holly families and certain plants in the Honeysuckle family have similar toxins		
Buttercup Family		
Plant	Toxin	Symptom
Larkspurs	Toxic alkaloids similar to aconitines, 14-deactylnudicauline, methylaconitine, and nudicauline	Nausea, vomiting, abdominal pain, blurred vision, dry mouth and dry skin. Restlessness, agitation, and dilated pupils that may last for more than twelve hours.
Black Hellebore, clematis or virgin bower, or leather flower, red baneberry, white baneberry, buttercups, crowfoot, blisterwort, tall buttercup, anemones, marsh marigolds, bulbous buttercup or St. Anthony's turnip, littleleaf	A mixtures of toxins, some are bufadienolides, saponins, and protoanemonin	Symptoms may be delayed and include pain in the mouth and abdomen, nausea, vomiting, cramps, diarrhea, visual disturbances, loss of appetite, and slow heart rate. It can also cause abortions in pregnant women. Clematis is also referred to as virgin bower, or leather flower, it

buttercup, sagebrush, and cursed buttercup		is more toxic with more of the same chemicals. It can cause blistering of the skin, vomiting of blood, weakness, and bloody diarrhea. Kidneys may be affected with painful urination, bloody urine and depletion in urine output, confusion, dizziness, fainting, and convulsions. Cooking deactivates the toxin. **Note:** Red and white baneberry causes circulatory failure.
Monkshood	Several diterpeniods, including aconitines, mesaconitine, napelline, and hypaconitine	Tingling and burning of the lips, tongue, mouth, and throat; headache; abdominal pain; excessive salivation; intense thirst;

		severe vomiting; diarrhea; cold feelings; slow heart rate; paralysis; confusion; restlessness; visual disturbances; convulsions; and delirium. Symptoms in severe cases are coma and death from asphyxiation and circulatory failure.
	Ginseng Family	
Plant	Toxin	Symptom
English ivy, Hercules club, and devils walkingstick	Teriterpene saponins	Vomiting, diarrhea, labored breathing, excitability, convulsions, and coma
	Holly Family	
Plant	Toxin	Symptom
English holly	Saponin and theobromine	Abdominal pain, nausea, vomiting, and drowsiness. Mild doses stimulate the central nervous system, but

		higher doses will depress it.
Honeysuckle Family		
Plant	Toxin	Symptom
Snowberry or waxberry, ghost-berry, and corpse-berry	Saponins, tannins, terpenes, coumarins, iridoids, and diterpenes	Vomiting, dizziness, mild sedation, gastrointestinal irritation, blood-stained urine, and a semi-comatose state

Cactus Family		
Plant	Toxin	Symptom
Peyote cactus	Peyotline, pellotine, anhalamine, anhalomineanine, anahalodine, and lophophorine	Nausea, chills, headache, severe abdominal pains, and vomiting, with terror, anxiety, dilated pupils, visual disturbances, hot-flushed face, relaxation of muscles, dizziness, decrease in heart rate, loss of sense of time and wakefulness

Carrot Family		
Plant	Toxin	Symptom
Poison hemlock, wild chervil, fools parsley, fernleaf, biscuitroot, waterparsnips, water parsley, hemlock, and waterdropwort or dead men's fingers	Coniine, gamma-coniceine, N-methylconiine, conhydrine, and pseudoconhydrine	Nausea, vomiting, salivation, abdominal pain, diarrhea, headache, dilated pupils, lack of coordination, confusion, sweating, difficulty breathing, coldness of extremities, drowsiness,

		fluctuation in blood pressure, rapid or irregular heartbeat, paralysis, convulsions, coma, and death from respiratory failure

Cashew Family		
Plant	Toxin	Symptom
Eastern poison ivy, Pacific poison ivy, Western poison ivy, poison oak, Atlantic poison oak, poison sumac, poison elder, staghorn sumac, and Florida poison tree	Catechol derivative, urushiols	Sap causes redness, itching, and burning of the skin. Small blisters may appear in a few hours or be delayed for as long as five days. Fruit and leaves cause upset stomach if eaten.

Conifer Family		
Plant	Toxin	Symptom
Yews, ponderosa pine, lodgepole pine, and loblolly pine	Isocupressic acid	Cause miscarriages

Cucumber Family		
Plant	Toxin	Symptom
Coastal manroot, bigroot, wild cucumber, balsampear, balsamapple, and bitter gourd	Tetracyclic triterpenes—cucurbitacins, abortifacients, alkaloids, and momordin	Chest pains, chest tightness, shortness of breath, restlessness, low blood pressure, internal bleeding from the loss of blood clotting function, and death. Seeds cause vomiting and diarrhea.

Cycad Family		
Plant	Toxin	Symptom
Cycad, commonly called sago palm	Beta-methylamino-L-alanine (BMAA), a neurotoxin and carcinogen	Affects nerves and spinal cord. Produces amyotrophic lateral sclerosis, Parkinson's disease and Lou Gehrig's disease.

Note: Cycasin and macrozamin are carcinogenic.

Dogbane Family		
Plant	Toxin	Symptom
Oleander, yellow oleander, yellow allamanda, or golden trumpet, and Indian hemp	Cardenolide oleandrin, several resins and glycosides, cymarin, apocannoside, and cyannocannoside	Nausea, severe vomiting, stomach pain, dizziness, slow pulse, irregular heartbeat, dilated pupils, bloody diarrhea, drowsiness, coma, possible respiratory paralysis, and death

Note: Oleander is the most dangerous because it causes bloody diarrhea.

Fern Family		
Plant	Toxin	Symptom
Bracken fern, horse tails, cloak fern, sensitive fern, and male fern	Some of the toxins include thiaminase-1(vitamin B_1), astragalin, isoquercetin, pterosides, pterosins, fumeric, succinic, shikimic acid, braxin A_1 and A_2 ptaquiloside, and d-econdysone. There are other toxins present, but I was unable to locate all of them.	Abdominal cramps, vomiting, diarrhea, and cancers of the bladder, esophagus, stomach, and liver. Acute hemorrhagic disease may develop.

Figwort and certain plants in the Lily family have similar toxins		
Figwort Family		
Plant	Toxin	Symptom
Purple foxglove	Several digitaloids, including digitoxin and digitalis	Nausea, vomiting, abdominal cramps, diarrhea, severe headache, irregular heartbeat, and tremors. Severe cases will produce convulsions and death. If the plant is served raw in a salad it may produce pain in the mouth and throat.
Lily Family		
Plant	Toxin	Symptom
Star of Bethlehem	Contains more than eight cardenolide toxins. Bulbs contain cardiac glycosides of digitalis.	Abdominal cramps, diarrhea slow or irregular heartbeat, and death
European lily of the valley	Contains more than twenty digitalis, like cardiac glycosides, convallatoxin, convallarin, convallamarin,	Burning pain in the mouth and throat, heavy salivation, nausea, vomiting, abdominal pain, cramping,

	asparagine, and volatile oils and resins	diarrhea, headache, dilated pupils, cold and clammy skin, dazedness, and slow, irregular heartbeat. The condition of the heart in this condition may sometimes lead to coma and death from heart failure.

Note: The foxglove flower produces blossoms in colors other than purple. The toxins directly influence the muscles of the heart.

Fumitory Family		
Plant	Toxin	Symptom
Bleeding hearts, Dutchman's breeches, squirrel corn, turkey corn, Pacific bleeding hearts, and showy	Isoquinoline alkaloids, aporphine, protoberberine, and protopine	Trembling, agitation, heavy salivation, vomiting, diarrhea, convulsions, tenseness of muscles, difficulty breathing, and prostration. Physical contact with plants may cause skin irritations.

Grass family and Morning Glory family have related toxins		
Grass Family		
Plant	Toxin	Symptom
Wild grasses, rye, durum wheat, and flowers of sorghum.	Ergot fungus and lysergic acid compounds	Intoxication, mild diarrhea, psychosis, and finally, dry gangrene of lower extremities
Morning Glory Family		
Plant	Toxin	Symptom
Morning glory, beach morning glory, granny vine, heavenly blue, pearly gates, flying saucer's wedding bells, Summer skies, and blue star	Ergot fungus and lysergic acid compounds	Intoxication, mild diarrhea, psychosis, and finally, dry gangrene of lower extremities

Heather Family		
Plant	Toxin	Symptom
Japanese pieris, rhododendrons, and azaleas	Grayanotoxins	Burning sensation in the mouth, watery eyes, salivation, runny nose, vomiting, abdominal pain, headache, prickly skin,

		muscular weakness, slow heart rate, fluctuating blood pressure from low to high, and paralysis
Sheep laurel, Mountain laurel, alpine laurel, and Labrador tea	Diterpene and acetylandromedol	These plants are more toxic. The additional symptoms are watering of the mouth, eyes, and nose; loss of appetite; repeated swallowing; drowsiness; convulsions; weakness; and difficulty breathing. Severe dosage will produce progressive paralysis of the limbs followed by coma and death.

Hemp Family		
Plant	Toxin	Symptom
Marijuana	Toxic resins that include tetrahydrocannabinol (THC)	Smoking marijuana causes throat irritation, coughing, dry mouth, eye irritation, nausea, and vomiting. Heavy concentrated doses may cause confusion, depression, paranoia, panic, memory loss, rapid heartbeat, high blood pressure, psychosis, and coma.

Honeysuckle, Rose, and Wild Cherry families and certain plants in the Pea family are composed of cyanide		
Honeysuckle Family		
Plant	Toxin	Symptom
Red elderberry, black elderberry, and blue elderberry	Cyanide	Diarrhea, speech problems, minor problems with memory, girdle pain, and delayed paralysis

Rose Family		
Plant	Toxin	Symptom
Apricots, peaches, plums, cherries, jet beads, saskatoon, serviceberry, mountain ashes, rowans, hawthorns, firethorns, cotoneasters, cherry laurel, Carolina laurel, and laurel cherry	Cyanide	Difficulty breathing, inability to speak, twitching, and spasms. Severe cases may result in a coma, followed by death.
Wild Cherry Family		
Plant	Toxin	Symptom
Chokecherry, black cherry, bitter cherry, and pin cherry	Cyanide	Anxiety, confusion, dizziness, headache, vomiting, smell of bitter almonds on the breath or vomit, difficulty breathing, fluctuations in blood pressure and heart rate, and kidney failure

Pea Family		
Plant	Toxin	Symptom
Bird-of-paradise, garden vetch, and winter vetch.	Cyanogenic glycoside, vicianine, and hydrocyanic acid. Toxic amino acids of beta-cyanoalanine and beta-aminopropionitrile	Rapid, difficult breathing; excitability; and restlessness. Severe-case symptoms are prostration, convulsions, coma, and death.

Note: Ripen fruit in wild cherry families is not toxic, while the other remaining plant parts including unripen fruit are toxic.

Iris Family		
Plant	Toxin	Symptom
Irises	Fresh plants have triterpene-aldehyde. Stored plants have alpha and gamma-iron.	Abdominal pain, nausea, vomiting, diarrhea, and fever

Lily Family		
Plant	Toxin	Symptom
Glory lily and autumn crocus	Colchicine and colchiceine	Symptoms are delayed from one hour up to forty-eight hours. There is intense burning of the mouth and throat, intense thirst, nausea,

		violent vomiting, severe abdominal pain, profuse and persistent diarrhea, shock from fluid loss, kidney damage, blood-stained urine, convulsions, coma, and death. Hair loss may result after two weeks of swallowing the toxic tea.
Snowdrop and daffodils	Amaryllidaceaen alkaloids with lycorine and galanthamine, and narcissine	Dizziness, abdominal pain, persistent vomiting, and diarrhea. Heavy doses will cause convulsions and death. Daffodils bring occasional diarrhea.
Aloes or aloe vera	Barbaloin and chrysophanic	Delayed symptoms from six to twelve hours. Symptoms are diarrhea from an irritated colon and possible irritation to the kidneys.

Green false hellebore and California false hellebore	Jervine, germidine, germitrine, veratroidine, veratrosine, and veratramine	Burning of the mouth and throat, upper abdominal pain, excessive salivation, vomiting, diarrhea, sweating, blurred vision, hallucinations, headache, general paralysis, and spasms. Severe cases have shallow breathing, irregular heart rate, low body temperature, seizures, and death.
Meadow death camas, foothill death camas, nuttalls death camas, pine barren death camas, wavy leaf soap plant, Western feather bells or mountain bells, and orchid	Zygacine, zygadenine, iso- and neogermidine, and protoveratridine	Burning of the mouth, numbness of the lips and mouth, excessive salivation, thirst, headache, confusion, dizziness, nausea, persistent vomiting, diarrhea, muscular weakness, slow and irregular heartbeat, low blood pressure,

		and low body temperature. Severe-case symptoms are difficulty breathing, seizures, coma, and death.

Lobelia Family		
Plant	Toxin	Symptom
Cardinal flower and Indian tobacco	Lobeline, lobelamine, and pyridine	Nausea, vomiting, salivation, abdominal pain, diarrhea, sweating, dilated pupils, lack of coordination, confusion, paralysis, low body temperature, low blood pressure, and fast, irregular heartbeat. Severe cases have convulsions, coma, and death.

Mahogany Family		
Plant	Toxin	Symptom
Chinaberry tree	Meliatoxins	Delayed symptoms: lack of coordination, confusion, and stupor. Severe-case symptoms are stomach pain, diarrhea, vomiting, difficulty breathing, convulsions, paralysis, and death.

Mezereum Family		
Plant	Toxin	Symptom
Daphnes	Daphnane, daphnin, daphnetin, and mezerein	Painful blisters of the lips, mouth, and throat, with salivation, thirst, and inability to eat. Irritated digestive tract, vomiting, bloody diarrhea, weakness, and headache. Severe-case symptoms are delirium, convulsions, coma, and death.

Milkweed Family		
Plant	Toxin	Symptom
Milkweeds	Galitoxins, cardioactive cardenolides, and steroidal glycosides that contain saponin	Dermatitis, depression, weakness, staggering, prostration, titanic seizures, labored breathing, high body temperature, dilated pupils, coma, and death.

Mistletoe Family		
Plant	Toxin	Symptom
Mistletoe and European mistletoe	Phoratoxin, polypeptide, and lectin	Minor abdominal pain and diarrhea

Moonseed Family		
Plant	Toxin	Symptom
Moonseed	Isoquinoline alkaloids with dauricine	Arrhythmias and seizures

Mulberry Family		
Plant	Toxin	Symptom
Edible fig and fiddle leaf fig	Ficin, ficusin, and 8-methoxypsoralen	Contact dermatitis and photodermatitis

Nightshade Family		
Plant	Toxin	Symptom
Angel's trumpet, Jerusalem cherry, belladonna or deadly nightshade, black henbane, tobacco, jimson weed, sacred thorn apple, desert thorn apple, prickly burr, and black nightshade	Solanine, dulcamarine, hyoscyamine, scopolamine, atropine, and nicotine	Dilated pupils, blurred vision, abdominal pain, flushing, dryness of skin and mucous membranes, hallucinations, headache, intense thirst, and nausea

Olive Family		
Plant	Toxin	Symptom
European privet, California privet, and Japanese privet	Iridoids	Severe gastrointestinal irritation, with vomiting, diarrhea, and convulsions

Pea Family		
Plant	Toxin	Symptom
Rosary pea	Abrin	Nausea, vomiting, diarrhea, severe abdominal pain, dilated pupils, ulceration and

		bleeding of the mouth and digestive tract, loss of intestinal function, and liver damage
Bird-of-paradise	Tannins	Nausea, vomiting, and diarrhea
Lupines	Sparteine, anagyrine, and lupanine	Vomiting, excessive salivation, nausea, dizziness, headache, abdominal pain, slow breathing, and slow heart rate
Flowering garden sweetpea, wild peas, wild lathyrus, caley pea, hoary pea, perennial pea, tiny pea, and flat pea	Lathyrogens and beta-aminopropionitrile	Lathyrism
Wisteria vine and black locust tree	Mixtures of lectins, agglutinins including isolectins	Nausea, abdominal pains, headache, dizziness, vomiting, and mild diarrhea

Golden chain tree	Quinolizidine alkaloids of cytisine	Rapid vomiting
Milk vetches and locoweeds	Selenium, aliphatic nitro-compounds, toxic indolizidin, alkaloid-swainsonine, glycoside of nitropropanol, and miserotoxin	Respiratory paralysis, huskiness of voice, and coughing
Showy rattlebox, false poinciana, and sesbane	Monocrotaline, spectabiline, retusine, retusamine, anacrotine, and nilgirine	Abdominal pain, nausea, vomiting, diarrhea, and loss of appetite
Scotch broom, Spanish broom, greenweeds, Kentucky coffee tree, mescal bean or Texas mountain laurel, and frijolito	Sparteine, isospartiene, and cytisine	Nausea, vomiting, dizziness, headache, and abdominal pain

Pink Family		
Plant	Toxin	Symptom
Corn cockle	Githagoside and other triterpenoid saponins	Drowsiness, yawning, diarrhea, vomiting, weakness, and weight loss

Pokeweed Family		
Plant	Toxin	Symptom
American pokeweed	Phytolaccatoxin and aglycone phytolaccagenin	Abdominal cramps, persistent vomiting, and diarrhea

Poppy Family		
Plant	Toxin	Symptom
Celandine, opium poppy, and bloodroot	Isoquinoline alkaloids consisting of coptisine, chelidonine, and berberine	Drowsiness, headache, and salivation
Opium poppy	Isoquinoline alkaloids consisting of morphine, codeine, papaverine, and various other toxins	Restlessness, excessive salivation, loss of appetite, stupor, and shallow, slow breathing
Bloodroot	Sanguinarine, chelerythrine, and resins	Vomiting, diarrhea, fainting, shock, coma, and death

Spurge Family		
Plant	Toxin	Symptom
Castor bean	Ricin	Burning in the mouth and throat, vomiting, severe stomach pain, diarrhea, thirst, prostration, headache, dizziness, lethargy, impaired vision, rapid heartbeat, and convulsions. Symptoms that may result within two to five hours are retinal hemorrhaging, internal bleeding, and fluid buildup in the digestive tract and lungs. The liver and kidneys will begin to deteriorate. Death usually occurs in twelve days from kidney failure.
Christ plant	Euphorbol	Severe irritations in the mouth and digestive tract
Garden croton	Crotonide, crotonic acid, crotin, and 12-O-	Dermatitis and diarrhea

	tetradecanoylphorbol-13-acetate	
Tungoil tree	Esters of 16-hydroxphorbol	Nausea, severe stomach pain, vomiting, and diarrhea

Verbana Family		
Plant	Toxin	Symptom
Lantana, red sage, and yellow sage	Lantadene	Weakness, lethargy, vomiting, diarrhea or constipation, loss of appetite, difficulty walking, and visual disturbances

Yew Family		
Plant	Toxin	Symptom
Yews	Taxol and taxine	Dry throat, nausea, vomiting, dizziness, dilated pupils, diarrhea with acute abdominal pain, and irregular heartbeat

You will notice that all poisonous teas made from most of the plants listed in the table will cause gastritis, which should be the first indicator in determining if you have swallowed a plant toxin. More severe symptoms are seizures and a coma. Plants in the buckthorn, conifer cycad, honeysuckle, rose, moonseed, mulberry, and nightshade families, and certain plants of the pea family, do not produce vomiting, nausea, and diarrhea for everyone. Plants in the arum, grape, beech, barberry, and cashew families (of poison ivies), milkweed, mulberry, and monkshood in the buttercup family, have toxins in the sap on their surfaces that cause skin dermatitis and eye irritations. Home manufacturers are not likely to use these because of the mouth swelling. That can be bad for business, because victims will be able to immediately determine something is in their food. Borage, beech, buttercup, wild cherry, lily pea, aster, fern, and spurge families will cause liver damage and cancers of the liver, esophagus, stomach, and bladder. Horse chestnut, carrot, dogbane, pea, and boxwood families have toxins that will cause respiratory and circulatory failure. Seizures, which are often referred to as convulsions, are cause by toxins in the buttercup, ginseng, boxwood, figwort, pea, lily, lobelia, mezereum, and olive families. If you desire bloody urine, try a toxic tea from the buttercup and honeysuckle families. Combine that with an extra cocktail made from a plant in the buttercup, dogbane, mezereum, pea, or cucumber family.

You will need to plan on a doggie bag if someone within your circle serves you a toxic tea from the buckthorn, buttercup, cashew, and poppy families, because the symptoms are delayed. Certain plants from the buttercup family will cause both bloody urine and bloody diarrhea. Honeysuckle also produces delayed paralysis! Interested in long-term care? Families of buckthorn, horse chestnut, carrot, heather, lobelia, mahogany, and pea will produce short-term or permanent and partial or complete paralysis depending on which plant toxin you are served. The cycad family is the only one that I found in the research that has toxins with a reputation for causing Parkinson's, and amyotrophic lateral sclerosis. The pea family will encourage you to control your insulin because it has a plant that can potentially cause type 1 diabetes. It will also tamper with your liver by causing veno-occlusive disease, referred to also as Budd-Chiari syndrome. Foxglove and moonseed families will interfere with your heart, creating sudden death (autoimmune myocarditis). The sudden change in your health will leave cardiac physicians scratching their heads! If you do not want to sleep for a while and, in some situations, sleep into death, do not allow anyone to serve you a toxic cocktail made from plants from the ginseng, honeysuckle, carrot, lily, rose, pea, lobelia, mezereum, milkweed, or poppy families, because the toxic tea will put its victim into a coma. Buttercup and conifer families have a reputation for causing miscarriages in pregnant mothers. Finally, toxic teas created using plants from the grass, morning glory, hemp, and nightshade families will leave you with short-term or long-term psychosis. Depending on the plant, amount of toxin, and length of time given, the victim will develop dry gangrene of the lower limbs that will have to be amputated. Physicians will search through all lab tests looking for an answer. There will be traces of LSD, leading doctors to think the patient was using drugs.

Chapter 5

Effects of Plant Poisoning

Digestion of food begins in the mouth, and food then travels through the esophagus into the stomach, where digestion continues. Food continues into the small intestines, where digestive enzymes, hormones, and bile from the gallbladder are combined with it to continue digestion. The liver is one of our major organs, and damage from plant and animal toxins can be deadly, because this organ performs many functions (Stanfordchildrens.org 2015).

Functions of the liver include producing cholesterol and special proteins that assist in carrying fats and proteins for blood plasma. It stores iron that it uses to make hemoglobin, which assists the red blood cells in carrying oxygen, and it regulates blood clotting. It produces immune components to combat infection and removes bacteria from the blood. It detoxifies and metabolizes toxins and then filters the blood of harmful toxins. It gets rid of bilirubin and aged red blood cells, or we would have jaundice. It produces bile and stores it in the gallbladder. The gall bladder releases bile into the small intestine as needed to break down fats and carry away harmful toxins and other wastes in the feces. It stores and releases glucose when needed for energy.

During digestion, a large percentage of ammonia is made in the small intestines and is absorbed back into the blood. The liver metabolizes the ammonia into urea, which is later filtered from the blood by the kidneys. The urea is then passed on to the bladder and is excreted from the body in the urine.

The body's response to any toxin is first to try to get rid of it, which is why most people will become nauseated and begin vomiting. Depending on the type of plant, the symptoms may include headaches, hallucinations, confusion, intoxication, weakness, loss of appetite, and abdominal pain or cramps. Once the liver cannot metabolize and get rid of the toxin, other symptoms may begin to appear, such as depression, loss of coordination, difficulty breathing, difficulty walking, and dilated pupils.

When the body is attacked with poisoning, the liver tries to do its job, but when there is an overload, as with toxic cocktails or toxic teas, the body's immune system is compromised. However, this system is designed to deal with bacteria, viruses, and toxins. Parts of this system include the tonsils and adenoids, lymph nodes, lymphatic vessels, thymus gland, spleen, appendix, Peyer's patches, and bone marrow (AIDS.gov 2015). This system is so effective that it knows when the body has been invaded by bacteria, viruses, parasites, transplanted tissue, transplanted organs, and toxins or poisoning. Each part has its own special function. It recognizes toxins as foreign antigens and goes through a process of producing antibodies to attack and get rid of them.

When a toxin is recognized by the immune system, it uses T-cells produced by the thymus gland to send out signals to build an attack system. T-cells help destroy cancer cells and infected cells. There are also B-cells, which are produced by lymphocytes in bone marrow and help fight bacteria and toxins. B-cells also use the signal sent out by T-cells to make antibodies to be released in all parts of the body to fight toxins. When body cells or tissues become invaded by toxins that cannot be recognized by the immune system, it decides that the cells are strange or unknown. It begins to treat them as foreign invaders and begins to attack. This is when an autoimmune disease develops. The type of autoimmune disease that develops will depend on which plant was used to make the toxic tea.

Chapter 6

Autoimmune Disease

For reasons that are mysterious to medical professionals, the immune system in certain individuals attacks its own cells, tissue, and organs, which is what occurs when an autoimmune disease has developed. The goal of the immune system is to produce antibodies made specifically to attack and destroy invaders when they enter the body, much in the same way our military stays alert and ready to attack invaders that threaten America. When an autoimmune disease has developed, the body's immune system gets tricked into thinking that its own cells are invaders. The immune system begins to make autoantibodies that attack and destroy what it is supposed to protect. In other words, the body turns on itself.

Which specific invader (drugs, germs, bacteria, or plant poison) is causing this disorder, what the cure or antidote is, what the origin of this invader is, and how it can be eradicated are the mysteries that repeatedly keep medical professionals at a loss for answers.

Autoimmune diseases are chronic and life threatening. The American Autoimmune Related Disease Association (AARDA) estimates that approximately fifty million Americans have an autoimmune disease. The National Institutes of Health (NIH) estimates that approximately 23.5 million Americans have an autoimmune illness. (AARDA 2013, 2014). Autoimmune disease is one of the top ten leading causes of death in female children and in women in all age groups under age sixty-four (Fairweather, Frisancho-Kiss, and Rose 2008). This rate is higher than heart disease, which is twenty-two million, and cancer, which is nine million. This heart-disease statistic may or may not include autoimmune myocarditis, which is an autoimmune heart condition. In America, autoimmune disease is the second leading cause of chronic illness. It is the third leading cause of Social Security disabilities. Approximately 9.8 million women are suffering with one of the following most common autoimmune diseases: Crohn's disease, Graves' disease, lupus, multiple sclerosis, psoriasis, rheumatoid arthritis, scleroderma, Sjogren's syndrome, type 1 diabetes, autoimmune myocarditis, and inflammatory bowel disease (AARDA 2013). This is not to say that men do not have autoimmune diseases—they do. The 22 percent of men that have autoimmune diseases are typically under the age of fifty, and they have a higher mortality rate because their immune systems are different and they do not respond as well as women to infection and trauma.

There is treatment for autoimmune diseases, but sadly, there is no cure. Many people are misdiagnosed, because the medical community is not adequately prepared for this drastic epidemic of plant poisoning. Therefore, it is hard for any medical physician to determine a diagnosis. This is confusing for physicians, suffering patients, and their families. More research and development is needed, especially for autoimmune diseases caused by plant poisoning.

The next part of this book will briefly describe each autoimmune disease as it relates to plant poisoning. The disease descriptions will include the physiological characteristics along with the plant and toxins involved, how they affect the body, and the symptoms as indicated by the research.

During the scope of my research, I found approximately ten autoimmune diseases or conditions that are disabling and can result in death, depending on the amount of toxic cocktail that certain individuals are administering to their victims in obscure ways. Those autoimmune diseases or conditions are amyotrophic lateral sclerosis (commonly called ALS), autoimmune myocarditis, type 1 diabetes, ergotism, psychosis, hyperaldosteronism, hepatotoxicity, cancers of the liver and esophagus, progressive paralysis, and neurolathyrism. There are other conditions that can result from being given toxic cocktails. There is scanty research indicating that lupus, an autoimmune disease, is caused by the toxin in raw alfalfa beans. The diseases mentioned in this book are ones that I found in the research that occurred most often. Coma and death can occur with any poison if enough is ingested.

Chapter 7

Amyotrophic Lateral Sclerosis

The sago palm plant originated in southern Japan and is now grown as an ornamental plant worldwide (Mason.gmu.edu 2015). In the United States, it grows in Alabama, Florida, Georgia, Louisiana, Mississippi, Southern California, South Carolina, southern North Carolina, and Texas. It is one of the most deadly plants. It contains three toxins—cycasin, BMMA (B-methylamino-L-alanine), and macrozamin—in the entire plant (Williams 2012). BMMA is a neurotoxin that affects nerves and can also cause seizures, dizziness, and severe headaches. Cycasin is both a carcinogen and a mutagen, which is a chemical that changes the genetic material in a cell and can possibly be carcinogenic. Macrozamin is also a carcinogen. A combination of all three chemicals working together creates a dangerous combination of toxins.

Cycasin poisoning can cause ALS, Parkinson's, prostate cancer, and fibrolemellar hepatocellular carcinoma, which is cancer of the liver. This poisoning has been found on the island of Guam, where sago palm is prepared and used as a food source. ALS is a disease of specific parts of the nervous system that are responsible for controlling voluntary muscle movement. There is a lack of muscle nourishment as well as a loss of signals the nerves send to muscles. There is also side damage to the spinal cord, which includes hardening. This can, in some cases, cause progressive paralysis. Death usually occurs in three to five years from respiratory problems. However, there are some individuals who have lived for years. Involuntary muscles that control the heartbeat, gastrointestinal functions, bowel movements, bladder excretion, and sexual functions are not affected by ALS. Hearing, vision, touch, and academic ability remain functional, but the muscles of the face, mouth, and throat are affected by the disease. There is also muscle twitching and cramping because the deteriorating nerves are abnormally sensitive. ALS reveals itself with weakness in an arm or leg and difficulty using the affected arm or leg (Amyotrophic lateral sclerosis 2002). There may also be difficulty in controlling speech or in swallowing. It will usually spread from one part of the body over to the adjacent side, such as from one arm over to the next arm or from one leg over to the next leg. A cane and exercise may be helpful at the beginning, but the disease may progress to the point at which using a cane or exercise will be impossible. Once it has progressed to this point, your health-care provider will probably run a series of tests to verify this condition. Doctors cannot reverse the disease; they can only treat the symptoms. According to my research, one drug has been approved by the Food and Drug Administration that may help with this disease. It is riluzole, brand name Rilutek.

Other diseases that resemble ALS include different forms of muscular dystrophy, such as spinal-bulbar muscular dystrophy, adult-onset spinal muscular atrophy, and myasthenia, which is a nerve-to-muscle condition that is typically caused by tumors pressing on the spinal cord or brain stem.

Chapter 8

Autoimmune Myocarditis

Autoimmune myocarditis is inflammation of the inner, thick muscle of the heart, called the myocardium, and necrosis of myocytes. Necrosis of myocytes is death or wasting away of cells in the heart that are adjacent to the myocardium. Myocarditis has many causes, but for the sake of this book, I will focus on autoimmune myocarditis, because it can be caused by exposure to toxic agents. Therefore, it is also referred to as toxic myocarditis.

The purple foxglove flower is often used by individuals seeking to do harm or gain control over others. This flower contains the toxic cardiac glycosides digoxin and digitoxin. Foxglove has medicinal uses that were initially introduced into the practice of cardiac medicine beginning in

1775 by several physicians. Several derivatives have been isolated from the plant to treat conditions of the heart. The side effects of the drug were realized during the eighteenth century. Physicians discovered that the drug was not as effective as once believed (Chopra and Nanda, 2013). They found out that overuse of the drug causes an increase in heart failure as well as a decrease in the ability to exercise. It has been used as a home remedy to treat dropsy, which is edema. It helps eliminate excess fluid until it has been consumed too long; then death eventually occurs. Autoimmune myocarditis initially reveals itself with an irregular heartbeat.

According to Stine and Brown (2015), the cardiac glycoside toxins interfere with the levels of sodium, calcium, and potassium in the heart muscle. Impaired function in the heart muscle can lead to congestive heart failure, in which the heart is unable to pump blood to tissues all over the body. If it is caught early, it can be repaired; if it is not, it can be deadly. People with congestive heart failure will suffer from fatigue, swelling in the lower limbs, and hypertrophy of the heart muscle. Swelling is referred to as edema, which is an accumulation of fluid in body tissues. Hypertrophy of the heart is an enlargement of the left ventricle, the main pumping chamber.

The Myocarditis Foundation (2015) has indicated that most individuals with myocarditis do not have symptoms and have not been diagnosed. They have further indicated that the most common symptom is shortness of breath during exercise or upon exertion. Shortness of breath may not present itself until nighttime, when the individual may be forced to sit up just to breathe. Other symptoms, as mentioned earlier, are abnormal heart rate, fatigue, chest pain or chest pressure, swelling or edema in the lower extremities, lightheadedness, and, in some individuals, sudden loss of consciousness. It would be worthwhile to perform a toxicology screening on all healthy professional athletes when they suddenly began to experience heart problems to prevent mysterious deaths from sudden heart attacks.

Chapter 9

Bloody Diarrhea

The garden croton, spurges, and daphnes are grown in the home both as indoor plants and as outside ornamental yard plants. They have toxins so toxic that if they come in contact with the skin and if the oil or sap is ingested, they will cause you to become ill (Keeler and Tu 1991). Oil from the garden croton causes delirium, gastroenteritis, cyanosis, bloody diarrhea, and respiratory failure. Four seeds can cause death. Skin contact with the sap can cause a burning pain and an erythematous papulovesicular rash, which is a blistery rash similar to chicken pox. Croton-seed poisoning by swallowing causes a hot, burning pain in the mouth, throat, and stomach (Karmakar 2007). There is also extra saliva, nausea, vomiting, abdominal pain, bloody diarrhea, exhaustion, failure of the circulatory and respiratory systems, and death.

Toxins in the daphne plant are mezerein, daphnetoxin, and 12-hydroxydaphnetoxin (Barceloux 2008). Mezerein has been found to be a second-stage tumor producer. Consuming poison from this plant has caused nausea, vomiting, abdominal pain, and diarrhea; in some cases there is bloody urine as well as bloody diarrhea.

According to Keeler and Tu (1991), spurges contain the carcinogenic toxins diterpene esters. However, they may not be used to make a tea because of the amount of thorns that are on the plant, making it difficult to harvest; therefore, you are unlikely to ingest the toxin. Remember, anything is possible; evil people out to make easy, tax-free money will use what is available.

There are numerous toxins in another beautiful yard flower: oleander; some familiar toxins are oleandrin, digitoxigenin, and neriantin. There are others with limited cardiac activity (Barceloux 2008). According to Grossberg and Fox (2007) and Hayes (2008), when those toxins are given regularly, they have the potential to do harm. When they are initially swallowed, nausea and abdominal pain is experienced, followed by bloody diarrhea that progresses into cardiac arrhythmias, slow heart rate, heart failure, unconsciousness, coma, and death.

The beautiful oleander flower is considered one of the most poisonous plants in the world. However, it has medicinal uses in the correct dosage and has been used to control an irregular heart rate; reduce fluid buildup, or edema, in the body; treat scabies, hemorrhoids, and parasites; and increases blood flow to the kidneys (Grossberg and Fox 2007).

Chapter 10

Cyanide Poisoning

Cyanide is a compound of cyanogenic glycosides that has medicinal uses in cancer treatment when properly used by medical professionals. Cyanide has become a homicidal tool for those who intend to do harm and is easily manufactured by those individuals who have chosen to do harm to others. A selection of plant parts from a variety of fruit plants is used to create a toxic cocktail of cyanide poisoning, because they contain hydrocyanic acid. Amygdalin is the major cyanogen. It is processed from the bark, stem, leaves, seeds, flowers, buds, and roots of the chokecherry, cherry, apricot, apple, peach, plum, crabapple, elderberry, and untreated bitter almond. The poisonous tea is made by crushing the fruits with their internal seeds, along with the bark, stem, leaves, buds, and flowers, and in some instances the roots (Keeler and Tu 1991). This mixture is soaked in water to leach out the cyanide—a very easy process, because cyanide is water soluble. Eating the ripe fruit without the seeds is harmless. Sometimes when we eat an apple, a couple of seeds may be accidentally swallowed. There is little danger of getting cyanide poisoning in these cases, because the liver is able to detoxify a minimal amount of cyanide poisoning.

Harm resulting from consuming cyanide tea depends on the size of the individual as well as the amount and frequency of drinking or eating the poison. According to Keeler and Tu (1991), acute cyanide poisoning can result in death, because it mostly affects the nervous, circulatory, and respiratory systems. It deprives the body of oxygen (Gardner and McGuffin 2013). It causes short-term increases in blood pressure and heart rate. Symptoms of mild poisoning include an unsteady gait or walk, feelings of stiffness in the lower limbs and hips, headache, drowsiness, speech difficulties, and girdle pain (pain in the lower back and in one or both hip joints). Other symptoms of cyanide poisoning may include hyperventilation, feelings of anxiety, confusion, inability to speak, vertigo, headache, nausea, vomiting, weakness, violent seizures, and collapse, which may be followed by a coma (Goetz 1985). A large overdose can result in death from within a few minutes to as long as one hour.

Chapter 11

Type 1 Diabetes

Type 1 diabetes is an autoimmune disease that occurs because of beta-cell failure in the pancreas. With beta-cell failure, the pancreas stops producing insulin. Medical professionals believe that this type of diabetes occurs because it develops from environmental factors in genetically predisposed individuals. There is an autoimmune series of actions in the body that mistakenly destroys insulin-producing cells also referred to as beta cells, inside the pancreas. The function of beta cells is to produce, store, and release insulin, which is a hormone that reduces blood glucose concentration by converting glucose into energy.

Poisonous teas or toxic cocktails made from plants from the pea family can be harmful. Depending on the dosage, they can be deadly. The black locust tree and the beautiful flowering wisteria vine contain toxic lectins, which are poisonous plant proteins that bind carbohydrates to cells and interfere with food protein synthesis. Another toxin group is agglutinins, which cause agglutination, or clotting of red blood cells. This clotting can produce a stroke. The wisteria vine also contains robin, which causes disturbances in the glycogen levels in the liver and muscle cells. With small, frequent doses, type 1 diabetes can develop, because the toxins have caused the beta cells to become dysfunctional. Therefore, the pancreas cannot produce insulin. Two other plants contain the same toxins and are deadly: the mistletoe and the rosary pea. Hopefully, no one will use them. Other symptoms that can develop as a result of ingesting a larger dose of the toxins are severe intoxication, nausea, vomiting that may include blood, and bloody diarrhea. A loss of fluids from the vomiting and diarrhea can produce hypovolemic shock, electrolyte disturbance, coma, and death. These symptoms may be delayed for as long as twenty-four hours after consuming the toxins.

The cycasin toxin from the sago palm changes in the body into another toxic chemical, methylazoxymethanol (MAM) that damages pancreatic islet of Langerhans cells. This can also cause type 1 diabetes (Williams 2012).

Chapter 12

Ergotism and Psychosis

Ergotism is a condition in which victims suffer severe cases of gangrene, leading to loss of limbs. It is produced by ergot, which is a fungus, Claviceps purpurea that grows as a parasite, mainly on rye and various grasses, such as Dallas grass. Different species grow on the floral parts of sorghum and on leaves and roots of morning glory (Santa Ana III 1997).

Ergotism has been referred to as "St. Anthony's fire," "the holy fire," and "St. Vitus's dance." St Anthony's fire occurred in 1951 in a village called Pont Saint Esprit. Approximately twenty people in this village were poisoned by the ergot fungus in the rye flour that they had used in cooking their bread. The symptoms they experienced included vomiting, hallucinations, running in the streets, and burning sensations in their limbs.

Ergot is presently cultivated for its medicinal uses in treating hormone-dependent tumors such as breast cancer, psychosis, Parkinson's disease, and strengthen the immune system. Unfortunately, in the hands of evil practitioners, ergot alkaloids produce gangrene of the lower extremities, because the alkaloids affect circulation and neurotransmission. Victims will experience intoxication when they initially swallow the toxins. If victims are given repeated doses, other symptoms that will slowly develop are a burning sensation in the limbs, hallucinations, irrational behavior, unconsciousness, and death.

In June of 2013, the European Union (EU) restricted the use of medications containing ergot derivatives because of the drug risks. There are five ergot derivatives: dihydroergocristine, dihydroergocryptine with caffeine, dihydroergotoxine, nicergoline, and dihydroergotamine. The drug derivatives can potentially cause three serious side effects. First, fibrosis can develop, which is thickening and scarring of connective tissue. Second, spasms or involuntary contractions can occur in the walls of arteries, veins, and internal organs. Finally, blood circulation can be obstructed, which decreases the ability of the circulatory system to supply blood to all parts of the body, especially lower limbs, leading to dry gangrene.

Heat destroys most teas produced by practitioners of plant poisoning, but according to clinical research, ergot alkaloids are not destroyed by heat. The ergot fungus can affect every system in the human body. The nervous and cardiovascular systems are harmed the most. It is dangerous to pregnant mothers, because it will cause the fetus to abort. Patients may lose fingers, toes, and complete limbs to dry gangrene that is caused by the ergot alkaloid ergotamine. Several ergot alkaloids are present in the fungus and are responsible for different symptoms. One series of alkaloids is lysergic acid hydroxyethylamide (LSD), which can interfere with the dopamine activity in the brain, causing confusion, delusions, and hallucinations (Matossian 1989). This may be followed by short-term as well as long-term psychosis. The fungus can be passed on in the mother's breast milk, which will poison the infant. This toxin has had medicinal uses in the past but has since been banned from usage because it can cause abortions as well as hemorrhaging.

Evil practitioners who are manufacturing homemade, poisonous teas or toxic cocktails are using the seeds, leaves, and roots of the morning-glory plant and flowers from infected sorghum for the ergot alkaloids. The toxins are strongest in the seeds of the morning glory. It grows in the wild and is also in many home gardens.

Chapter 13

Hyperaldosteronism

Hyperaldosteronism is a condition in which one or both adrenal glands secrete too much aldosterone. Aldosterone is a steroid hormone made by the adrenal glands. Based on research on Emedicine.medscape.com (2015), this condition causes too much sodium to be reabsorbed and the loss of too much potassium and hydrogen ions. One of the causes of hyperaldosteronism is ingestion of too much licorice.

Licorice comes from a perennial herb called wild licorice (Vizgirdas and Rey-Vizgirdas 2006). This plant contains glycyrrhizin, sugar, and other chemicals that have a variety of uses. It is used medicinally as a mild laxative to soothe irritated and inflamed mucous membranes of the mouth, and it is used as a sweetener to improve the taste of other drugs. It is used in creating desserts and to sweeten chewing tobacco. The root and aboveground runners have been processed into an herbal tea remedy and used to treat asthma, stomach ulcers, bronchitis, and urinary-tract infections. Medical researchers believe that glycyrrhizin is effective in fighting cancer. It was also used to treat problems of hepatitis (Kole et al. 2010). The use of glycyrrhizin tea has been limited because of the problems it causes with sodium and potassium (Williams 2012). It has toxic effects at higher doses. As it is reabsorbed in the body, it interferes with the enzyme in the kidneys that converts cortisol to cortisone. Decreased activity of this enzyme causes an increase of cortisol, which causes water and sodium to be retained and many potassium and hydrogen ions to be excreted by the kidneys. When this occurs for a long period of time, it causes an increase of blood pressure from the loss of potassium.

Chapter 14

Liver Damage (Hepatotoxicity)

The US Library of Medicine has stated that the liver is the largest organ in the body and a vital organ that we cannot live without (Nlm.nih.gov 2015). It aids in the digestion of fats, stores energy, and removes toxins. Like many other organs in our bodies, it can be compromised. Liver disease can occur from a variety of causes, and it is the fifth most common cause of death. In my research, toxic cocktails or poisonous teas, such as the tea from the lantana flower, can harm the liver. The lantana is a drought-resistant, pest-resistant, ornamental flower that is poisonous. Jamkhande, Tolsarwad, and Tidke (2013) indicated that the lantana flower contains toxins that can cause hepatotoxicity. Hepatotoxicity is chemically induced liver damage from hepatotoxins. Hepatotoxins are chemicals or drugs that cause damage to the liver. The lantana flower toxin is lantadene, which closely resembles cholesterol and is easily absorbed by the liver. Cholesterol and other chemicals from the blood are used by the liver to make bile acids.

Lantana toxins injure the bile canalicular membrane. The canalicular membrane lines the walls of the bile canaliculi, which are small bile vessels inside the liver that collect bile as it is produced by hepatocytes, special cells in the liver. According to Acamovic, Stewart, and Pennycott (2014), phylloerythrin, which is a metabolic product, is a photosensitive compound produced when chlorophyll is metabolized. It is combined in the liver with bile and is excreted out of the body in a healthy individual. Lantadene toxin prevents this from occurring. Instead, the toxin causes intrahepatic cholestasis, a condition in which the flow of bile from the liver is blocked. It prevents phylloerythrin and bile from being excreted. Another consequence of this is an excess buildup of bilirubin. Bilirubin is the yellow pigment in bile. It is a waste product from older red blood cells being replaced by new red blood cells. Bilirubin is what gives solid waste (feces) its brown color. A buildup of bilirubin causes jaundice in the body. Visible symptoms of jaundice include yellowing of the white part of the eyes as well as yellowing of the skin. This blockage also causes phylloerythrin to accumulate beneath the skin, causing photosensitization. This causes the skin to react to sunlight. Some individuals may develop a blistery skin rash after being exposed to sunlight. On the first day of swallowing lantana poisoning, there may be intoxication, a loss of appetite, sluggishness, partial paralysis, and bloody diarrhea. Haschek, Rousseaux, and Wallig (2013) suggest that, depending on the amount ingested, liver lesions can develop, as well as edema in the liver and in the gallbladder, enlarged kidneys, damage to the heart, pulmonary edema, and emphysema. Gross edema to lower limbs, followed by necrosis of the liver and death, can also occur. Lantana poisoning can be detected in the solid waste from the lower gastrointestinal tract.

According to Williams (2012) and Jamkhande, Tolsarwad, and Tidke (2013), the cycasin toxin from the cycad sago palm has the ability, in high doses, to cause liver failure as well as gastrointestinal irritation. It plays a very large role in causing cancers of the liver (Motulsky 1989).

Chapter 15

Liver and Esophageal Cancers

Cancer is one of life's worst enemies. As most of us are aware, cancers are masses of abnormal cells growing at different rates and possibly spreading to a variety of areas in the body. There are a number of different kinds of toxic cocktails that are sources of carcinogens. One is a poisonous tea made from bracken fern, a plant that is considered a weed by some and an ornamental plant by others. It is grown inside the home or in the yard. To humans, bracken fern is clastogenic, carcinogenic, and antithiaminic. The toxins are clastogenic because they have the potential to cause normal cells to develop mutations, cause chromosomes to break apart, and become deleted. They are carcinogenic because they cause cancer. They are antithiaminic because they destroy thiamine, Vitamin B_1. A deficiency of this vitamin can cause hemorrhaging (Somvanshi and Ravisankar 2004). The interaction that occurs between DNA and the toxin ptaquiloside causes esophageal carcinoma and gastric cancers, a variety of cancers in the third section of the small intestine (ileum) where it connects or meets the large intestine, and cancers of the urinary bladder. Its antithiaminic toxins degrade vitamin B_1.

According to Williams (2012), cycasin from the sago palm plant is responsible for causing not only autoimmune amyotrophic lateral sclerosis and Parkinson's disease but also cancer of the liver. The body's intestinal flora has the ability to change cycasin into a more toxic, carcinogenic compound, methylazoxymethanol (MAM), which causes cancer of the liver.

The American Indians used rhizomes and roots of the bracken fern for many medicinal purposes (Foster and Hobbs 2002): to treat a prolapsed uterus, to stimulate milk production in nursing mothers, and to treat chest pain, diarrhea, burns, and arthritis. A poultice was made and applied to the area with a homemade cloth bandage. A poultice is a moist paste made from the plant. It was later realized that those populations who used the plant for various food sources had high rates of stomach, liver, and esophageal cancers. Bracken fern exposure in humans has been linked to cancers of the esophagus in several parts of the world (Campo 2006). In Japan where consumption is high, fiddlehead ferns are boiled in water to remove some of the toxin, but that is not 100 percent effective. Eating the fiddleheads after this treatment is still a risk.

In animal studies in which domestic and laboratory animals were fed large quantities of bracken fern, severe poisoning occurred (Somvanshi and Ravisankar 2004). The animals suffered thiamine deficiency, acute hemorrhagic disease, carcinomas of the upper digestive tract, and hematuria in cows. Hematuria in cows is characterized by bloody urine with clots. According to Keeler and Tu (1991), consuming herbal teas created from plant parts from the garden croton causes esophageal cancers and nasopharyngeal carcinomas.

Chapter 16

Neurolathyrism and Progressive Paralysis

Neurolathyrism is a neurotoxic disease found in humans that reveals itself with spastic partial paralysis of the buttocks and lower limbs. The disease begins with cramping of the calf muscles, which seems to occur after exposure to cold, physical exhaustion, and infection. Further symptoms include the paralysis, the urgent and frequent need to urinate, weakness, and pain. Younger males in their twenties and thirties are more affected than females of any age or males over thirty. An aortic aneurysm can develop. Based on the work of Chang and Slikker (1995), this disease was previously known to Hippocrates, the father of medicine.

Neurolathyrism is caused by ingesting a toxin from the grass pea. This plant is recognized by many as the ornamental sweet pea. It is a cool-weather flower. The toxin is beta-oxalylamino-L-alamine (L-BOOAA) and is present in the seedlings, seeds, and seedpods. The toxin will cause the gluteus maximus, or buttocks, to waste away and appear flat. Paralysis occurs because the toxin causes irreversible damage. The nervous system and skeletal system are damaged. There are aortic abnormalities, the metabolism in the connective tissues is damaged, and glutamic acid is damaged. Glutamic acid is an amino acid that is produced in the brain and is a neurotransmitter. It is responsible for the transmission of nerve impulses in the body. Victims also suffer from narcolepsy, which is a neurological condition in which the brain cannot control or distinguish nightly sleep hours from daily wake hours (Offermanns and Rosenthal 2008). Individuals are likely to fall asleep spontaneously even if they have just had a restful night of sleep.

Glory lily and autumn crocus contain colchicine, a mitotic poison or spindle poison that produces delayed reactions. Research has indicated cases of people living for as long as eight days before dying. Bone-marrow studies that were performed two hours before death revealed a tremendous decrease in both white blood cells and red blood cells. There was an increase in immature leukocytes, because adult cells had left the bone marrow. Symptoms included vomiting, bloody diarrhea, blood in the urine, progressive paralysis, loss of hair, and evidence of polyneuritis. Polyneuritis is pain, numbness, and tingling in the limbs. Colchicine is slowly metabolized by the body. In autopsy exams, various tissue samples had indications of arrested metaphase, meaning that cell division had stopped in its fourth stage (there are seven stages of cell division). Those tissue samples came from the liver, lymph glands, spleen, intestinal glands, adrenal cortex, pancreas, pituitary gland, and kidneys.

Conclusion

My purpose for writing this book was because I had the desire to explain a secret black-market crime. A crime that I, along with close family members, was exposed to. My wish is that after reading this book you will have gained an understanding of plant poison and a deeper respect for human life, how special it is not only for you, but also for everyone. My life experiences caused me to become determined to research voodoo and an inquisitive thought behind how it is supposed to make anyone do what culprits want. This was a path that led me from the voodoo ceremonies in the West Indies to the ceremonies as they occurred in New Orleans.

You have found in this book some history of voodoo and the reason people began to use it. It is also my desire to make everyone aware of how the poison-making criminals are able to produce toxic cocktails, also referred to as poisonous teas; how these are made in their homes; how they are sold and distributed on the black market and, finally, how they are administered to their intended victims. You have also been presented with plant families, plant toxins, and the harm the toxins are capable of doing to the body. There is information on autoimmune diseases and the toxins that cause them to occur. Each disease has a brief description of how the toxins cause changes in the biological processes that we need to live healthy and independently.

My hope is that after reading this book, if you find yourself exposed to someone who desires to control or harm you with plant poisoning, you are not only able to protect yourself but also able to prove to authorities that it occurred. It has been my experience that people do not believe you when you tell them someone has given you poison. The culprit lies so well that it sounds truthful, and proper authorities will believe the criminal before they will believe you, even though you are the one who is ill and suffering. I would like to see laws implemented into the local and federal judicial system for manufactures of plant poisoning, and their clients with penalties in the form of prison sentences in the same manner as it is with those criminals who manufacture and sell heroin, cocaine, and other dangerous drugs. Plant poisoning is more dangerous, kills much faster than heroin or cocaine, and is intentionally administered to kill, or seriously harm people. More lives would be saved and an improvement in treating health related autoimmune diseases if the medical professionals would develop and implement toxicology screening during medical visit for those individuals whose health suddenly takes a turn for the worst. Poison manufactures are able to aggressively market their products by telling their clients that physicians cannot find the special product (toxin).

References

AARDA. 2013. "AARDA Applauds Fox Sports Supports for Selecting Johns Hopkins Medicine as a 2013 Partner Charity." http://www.aarda.org/autoimmune-information/autoimmune-statistics/aarda.

AARDA. 2014. "News Briefing for Autoimmune Disease Awareness Month 2014." http://www.aarda.org/news-briefing-for-autoimmune-disease-awareness-month-2014/.

Acamovic, Thomas, Colin S. Stewart, and T. W. Pennycott. 2004. Poisonous Plants and Related Toxins. Wallingford, UK: CABI Publishing.

AIDS.gov. 2015. "Immune System 101." https://www.aids.gov/hiv-aids-basics/just-diagnosed-with-hiv-aids/hiv-in-your-body/immune-system-101/.

Amyotrophic Lateral Sclerosis. 2002. "Amyotrophic Lateral Sclerosis, Lou Gehrig's Disease." Hathitrust. http://babel.hathitrust.org/cgi/pt?id=pst.000050363148;view=1up;seq=9.

Barceloux, Donald G. 2008. Medical Toxicology of Natural Substances: Foods, Fungi, Medicinal Herbs, Plants and Venomous Animals. Hoboken, NJ: John Wiley and Sons.

Campo, M. Saveria. 2006. Papillomavirus Research: From Natural History to Vaccines & Beyond. Wymondham, UK: Caister Academic Press.

Chang, Louis W., and William Slikker. 1995. Neurotoxicology. San Diego: Academic Press.

Chopra, H. K., and Navin C. Nanda. 2013. Textbook of Cardiology: A Clinical and Historical Perspective. New Delhi, India: Jaypee Brothers Medical Publishers.

Emedicine.medscape.com. 2015. "Hyperaldosteronism: Background, Pathophysiology, Etiology." http://emedicine.medscape.com/article/920713-overview.

Fairweather, DeLisa, Sylvia Frisancho-Kiss, and Noel R. Rose. 2008. "Sex Differences in Autoimmune Disease from a Pathological Perspective." American Journal of Pathology 173 (3): 600–609. doi:10.2353/ajpath.2008.071008.

Foster, Steven, and Christopher Hobbs. 2002. A Field Guide to Western Medicinal Plants and Herbs. Boston: Houghton Mifflin.

Gardner, Zoe, and Michael McGuffin. 2013. American Herbal Products Association's Botanical Safety Handbook. 2nd ed. New York: CRC Press.

Goetz, Christopher G. 1985. Neurotoxins in Clinical Practice. Jamaica, NY: Spectrum Publications.

Grossberg, George, and Barry Fox. 2007. The Essential Herb-Drug-Vitamin Interaction Guide: The Safest Way to Use Medications and Supplements Together. New York: Broadway Books.

Haschek, Wanda M., Colin George Rousseaux, and Matthew A. Wallig. 2013. Haschek and Rousseaux's Handbook of Toxicologic Pathology. Amsterdam: Academic Press.

Hayes, A. Wallace. 2007. Principles and Methods of Toxicology. 5th ed. Boca Raton, FL: CRC Press.

Jamkhande, Prasad G., Ganesh S. Tolsarwad, and Priti S. Tidke. 2013. "Herbal Hepatotoxicity: A Review on Phytochemical Induced Liver Injury." Journal of Applied Pharmaceutical Science 3 (8): S106–S110.

Karmakar, R. N. 2007. Forensic Medicine and Toxicology. 2nd ed. Kolkata, India: Academic Publishers.

Keeler, R. F., and Anthony T. Tu. 1991. Handbook of Natural Toxins: Toxicology of Plant and Fungal Compounds. Vol. 1. New York: Marcel Dekker.

Kole, Chittaranjan, Charles H. Michler, Albert G. Abbott, and Timothy Hall. 2010. Transgenic Crop Plants: Principles and Development. Vol. 1. New York: Springer Heidelberg Dordrecht.

Mason.gmu.edu. 2015. "Poison Project Page." http://mason.gmu.edu/~kholguin/projects/poison.html .

Matossian, Mary Allerton Kilbourne. 1989. Poisons of the Past. New Haven, CT: Yale University Press.

Motulsky, Arno G. 1989. Diet and Health. Washington, D.C.: National Academy Press.

Myocarditis Foundation. 2015. "Myocarditis Causes, Symptoms, Diagnosis and Treatment." http://www.myocarditisfoundation.org/about-myocarditis/.

Nlm.nih.gov. 2015. "Liver Disease: Medlineplus." https://www.nlm.nih.gov/medlineplus/liverdiseases.html.

Offermanns, Stefan, and Walter Rosenthal. 2008. Encyclopedia of Molecular Pharmacology. 2nd ed. New York: Springer-Verlag Berlin Heidelberg.

Pussa, Tonu. 2014. Principles of Food Toxicology. Boca Raton, FL: CRC Press.

Santa Ana, Rod. 1997. "Devastating Sorghum Disease Spreads to United States." Agrilife Today. http://today.agrilife.org/1997/03/27/devastating-sorghum-disease-spreads-to-united-states/.

Somvanshi, R., and R. Ravisankar. 2004. "Recent Advances in Bracken Fern Toxin Research." Natural Product Radiance 3 (4): 304–307.

Stanfordchildrens.org. 2015. "Default—Stanford Children's Health." http://www.stanfordchildrens.org/en/topic/default?id=anatomy-and-function-of-the-liver-90-P03069.

Stewart, Amy. 2009. Wicked Plants: The Weed That Killed Lincoln's Mother and Other Botanical Atrocities. Chapel Hill, NC: Workman Publishing.

Stine, Karen E., and Thomas Brown. 2015. Principles of Toxicology. 3rd ed. Boca Raton, FL: CRC Press.

Tallant, Robert. 1946. Voodoo in New Orleans. New York: Macmillan.

Turner, Nancy J., and P. von Aderkas. 2009. The North American Guide to Common Poisonous Plants and Mushrooms. Portland, OR: Timber Press.

Vizgirdas, Ray S., and Edna M. Rey-Vizgirdas. 2006. Wild Plants of the Sierra Nevada. Reno: University of Nevada Press.

Williams, Cheryll J. 2012. Medicinal Plants in Australia. Sydney: Rosenberg Publishing.

Wink, Michael, and Ben-Erik van Wyk. 2008. Mind-Altering and Poisonous Plants of the World. London: Timber Press.